Christmas, 2012

Dr. Miller-

Sure hope
you have an appeti-
for these "Brain" snacks
with no concerns / worries
about calories + fat ...
but instead provide an
opportunity for pleasure
+ growth ☺

Fondly,
Beth Hanna Dingle

.

Brain Snacks

Quotes to Nourish your Mind

Shelli K. Margheritis

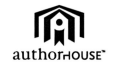

authorHOUSE™

1663 LIBERTY DRIVE, SUITE 200
BLOOMINGTON, INDIANA 47403
(800) 839-8640
WWW.AUTHORHOUSE.COM

First published by AuthorHouse 10/08/04

ISBN: 1-4184-9776-2 (sc)
ISBN: 1-4184-9775-4 (dj)

Library of Congress Control Number: 2004096896

Printed in the United States of America
Bloomington, Indiana

This book is printed on acid-free paper.

This book is dedicated to those who can read between the lines, therefore recognizing the power and enriched meaning of thought.

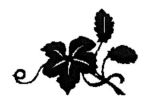

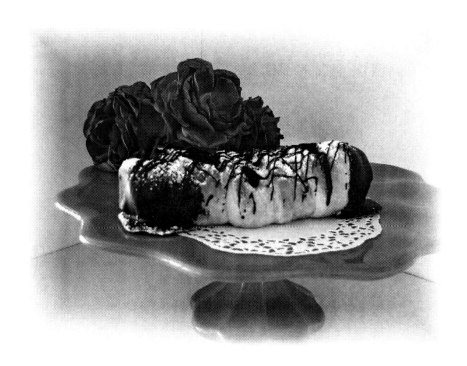

Table of Contents

Prologue

The definition of a quote is: To repeat or reproduce a passage, or a statement which is a reference from authority or from an example. In a nutshell, a quote can be a learning tool. Not all quotes are to be agreed upon, as they are quite simply statements made from other individuals' personal perceptions. However, within so many quotes there lies tremendous truth, reality, and inspiration.

Quotes have played an important role in all of our lives. We use them on a daily basis, sometimes without even recognizing it. Most of the time a quote can run through our thoughts without even having to be spoken. Haven't you ever questioned an individual's actions and heard yourself mumbling, "What goes around, comes around?" We have all used quotes at some point in our lives. They are a learned trait, and educators have used them for centuries as they are an extraordinary means in which to learn life lessons by.

Brain Snacks simply means food for your brain; that is what a quote is. Words are nourishment that feed your thoughts. Quotes enable you to ponder your own perspective, and determine your own creative definition. Enclosed within this book are just a few, or an appetizer if you will, of inspiring, eloquent, educational, profound, and thought-provoking quotes. Savor the knowledge!

Favorite Quotes
Words to live by

"Punctuality is the eloquence of Kings and Queens."
- Anonymous

"Being deeply loved by someone gives you
strength; loving someone
deeply gives you courage."
- Lao Tzu

"If you judge people, you have no time
to love them."
- Mother Theresa

"You are never given a wish without also being given
the power to make it come true. You may have to work
for it, however."
- Richard Bach

"The world is so fast that there are days when the person
who says it can't be done, is interrupted
by the person who is doing it."
- Anonymous

"Opportunities are usually disguised as hard work,
so most people don't recognize them."
- Ann Landers

"The grand essentials of happiness are: something to do, something to love, and something to hope for."
- Allan K. Chalmers

"Honesty is the first chapter in the book of wisdom."
- Thomas Jefferson

"Kindness is more important than wisdom, and the recognition of this is the beginning of wisdom."
-Theodore Isaac Rubin

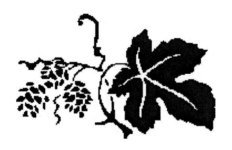

And……. an all time favorite …

"It is what it is."
-Anonymous

Words Flavored with Love and Life
Sugar n Spice, everything nice

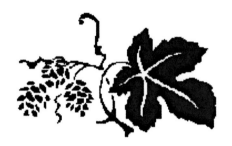

"Fear less, hope more;
Whine less, breathe more;
Talk less, say more;
Hate less, love more;
And all good things are yours."
- Swedish Proverb

"Learn from yesterday, live for today,
hope for tomorrow."
-Anonymous

"Some people weave burlap into the fabric of our lives,
and some weave gold thread. Both contribute to make
the whole picture beautiful and unique."
- Anonymous

"Life is like a beautiful melody, only the
lyrics are messed up."
- Anonymous

"Here is the test to find whether your mission on
Earth is finished: if you're alive, it isn't."
-Richard Bach

"Life consists not in holding good cards but in
playing those you hold well."
-Josh Billings

"The question is not whether we will die,
but how we will live."
- Joan Borysenko

"Do not dwell in the past, do not dream of the future,
concentrate the mind on the present moment."
- Buddha

"I still find each day too short for all the thoughts I
want to think, all the walks I want to take, all the
books I want to read, and all the friends I want to see."
- John Burroughs

"The purpose of life is a life of purpose."
- Robert Byrne

"Finish each day and be done with it. You have done
what you could; some blunders and absurdities have
crept in; forget them as soon as you can. Tomorrow is a
new day; you shall begin it serenely and with too high
a spirit to be encumbered with your old nonsense."
-Ralph Waldo Emerson

"All life is an experiment."
- Ralph Waldo Emerson

"It is not length of life, but depth of life."
-Ralph Waldo Emerson

"Never be bullied into silence. Never allow yourself to be made a victim. Accept no one's definition of your life; define yourself."
- Harvey Fierstein

"In three words I can sum up everything I've learned about life: it goes on."
- Robert Frost

"It's not your blue blood, your pedigree or your college degree. It's what you do with your life that counts."
- Millard Fuller

"Live as if you were to die tomorrow. Learn as if you were to live forever."
-Mahatma Gandhi

"What lies behind us and what lies ahead of us are tiny matters compared to what lives within us."
-Oliver Wendell Holmes

"The great use of life is to spend it for something that will outlast it."
-William James

"Believe that life is worth living and your belief
will help create the fact."
- William James

"This life is worth living, we can say,
since it is what we make it."
- William James

"The tragedy of life is not that it ends so soon, but that
we wait so long to begin it."
- W.M. Lewis

"Tell me not, in mournful numbers,
Life is but an empty dream!
For the soul is dead that slumbers,
and things are not what they seem.
Life is real! Life is earnest!
And the grave is not its goal;
Dust thou art; to dust returnest,
Was not spoken of the soul."
- Henry Wadsworth Longfellow

"Everything has been figured out, except how to live."
-Jean-Paul Sartre

"Live every day as if it were your last, because
one of these days, it will be."
-Jeremy Schwartz

"Not life, but good life, is to be chiefly valued."
- Socrates

"For some, life lasts a short while, but the
memories it holds last forever."
-Laura Swenson

"May you live every day of your life."
-Jonathan Swift

"You don't love a woman because she is beautiful, but
she is beautiful because you love her."
-Anonymous

"If you love somebody, let them go. If they return, they
were always yours. If they don't, they never were."
- Anonymous

"Love has nothing to do with what you are expecting to
get, it's what you are expected to give –
which is everything."
- Anonymous

"Love does not begin and end the way we seem
to think it does. Love is a battle, love is a war;
love is a growing up."
- James Baldwin

"Love takes off masks that we fear we cannot live
without and know we cannot live within."
- James Baldwin

"Love is the immortal flow of energy that nourishes,
extends and preserves. Its eternal goal is life."
- Smiley Blanton

"The best proof of love is trust."
- Joyce Brothers

"Sometimes the heart sees what is invisible to the eye."
- H. Jackson Brown Jr.

"We perceive when love begins and when it declines by
our embarrassment when alone together."
- La Bruyere

"Perfect love is rare indeed - for to be a lover will require that you continually have the subtlety of the very wise, the flexibility of the child, the sensitivity of the artist, the understanding of the philosopher, the acceptance of the saint, the tolerance of the scholar and the fortitude of the certain."
- Leo Buscaglia

"Where there is great love, there are always wishes."
- Willa Cather

"A relationship is like a rose, How long it lasts, no one knows; Love can erase an awful past, Love can be yours, you'll see at last; To feel that love, it makes you sigh, To have it leave, you'd rather die; You hope you've found that special rose, 'Cause you love and c are for the one you chose."
- Rob Cella

"Sympathy constitutes friendship; but in love there is a sort of antipathy, or opposing passion. Each strives to be the other, and both together make up one whole."
- Samuel Taylor Coleridge

"All thoughts, all passions, all delights, whatever stirs this mortal frame. All are but ministers of love and feed His sacred flame."
- Samuel Taylor Coleridge

"Friendship often ends in love;
but love in friendship - never."
-Charles Caleb Colton

"Woe to the man whose heart has not learned while
young to hope, to love - and to put its trust in life."
-Joseph Conrad

"Absence is to love what wind is to fire; it extinguishes
the small, it enkindles the great."
-Comte DeBussy-Rabutin

"Love builds bridges where there are none."
-R. H. Delaney

"We are all born for love. It is the principle
of existence, and its only end."
-Benjamin Disraeli

"Come live with me, and be my love, and we will some
new pleasures prove of golden sands, and crystal brooks,
with silken lines, and silver hooks."
-John Donne, "The Bait"

"You will find as you look back upon your life that the moments when you have truly lived are the moments when you have done things in the spirit of love."
-Henry Drummond

"Footfalls echo in the memory down the passage which we did not take towards the door we never opened into the rose-garden.
My words echo thus, in your mind."
-T. S. Eliot, "Four Quartets"

"The art of love … is largely the art of persistence."
-Albert Ellis

"All mankind love a lover."
-Ralph Waldo Emerson

"The hardest of all is learning to be a well of affection, and not a fountain; to show them we love them not when we feel like it, but when they do."
-Nan Fairbrother

"In love the paradox occurs that two beings become one and yet remain two."
-Erich Fromm

"Immature love says: 'I love you because I need you.'
Mature love says 'I need you because I love you.'"
-Erich Fromm

"Where there is love there is life."
-Mahatma Gandhi

"For it was not into my ear you whispered,
but into my heart. It was not my
lips you kissed, but my soul."
-Judy Garland

"Life without love is like a tree without blossoms or fruit."
-Kahlil Gibran, "The Vision"

"There is only one terminal dignity -- love."
-Helen Hayes

"The supreme happiness in life is the
conviction that we are loved."
-Victor Hugo

"The supreme happiness in life is the conviction that we
are loved -- loved for ourselves, or rather, loved in
spite of ourselves."
-Victor Hugo

"Looking back, I have this to regret, that too often when I loved, I did not say so."
-David Grayson

"Love can sometimes be magic. But magic can sometimes...just be an illusion."
-Javan

"The moment you have in your heart this extraordinary thing called love and feel the depth, the delight, the ecstasy of it, you will discover that for you the world is transformed."
-J. Krishnamurti

"The cure for all ills and wrongs, the cares, the sorrows and the crimes of humanity, all lie in the one word 'love.' It is the divine vitality that everywhere produces and restores life."
-Lydia Maria Child

"Treasure the love you receive above all. It will survive long after your good health has vanished."
-Og Mandino

"Do all things with love."
-Og Mandino

"The only abnormality is the incapacity to love."
-Anaïs Nin

"At the touch of love everyone becomes a poet."
-Plato

"We all suffer from the preoccupation that there exists
... in the loved one, perfection."
-Sidney Poitier

"There is no disguise which can hide love for long where it
exists, or simulate it where it does not."
-La Rochefoucauld

"To fear love is to fear life, and those who fear life
are already three parts dead."
-Bertrand Russell

"Tell me who admires you and loves you,
and I will tell you who you are."
-Charles Augustin Sainte-Beauve

"I have said nothing because there is nothing I can say
that would describe how I feel as perfectly
as you deserve it."
-Kyle Schmidt

"Love means never having to say you're sorry."
-Erich Segal

"Romeo, Romeo, wherefore art thou, / Romeo? /
Deny thy father, and refuse thy name..."
-William Shakespeare

"A very small degree of hope is sufficient
to cause the birth of love."
-Stendhal

"To fall in love is easy, even to remain in it is not
difficult; our human loneliness is cause enough. But
it is a hard quest worth making to find a comrade
through whose steady presence one becomes steadily
the person one desires to be."
-Anna Louise Strong

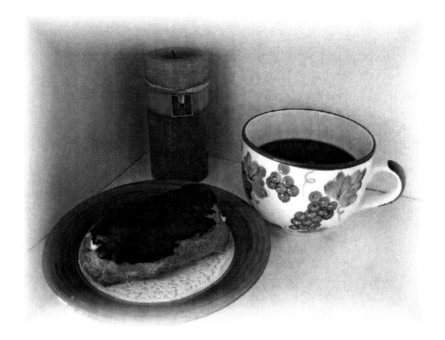

The Rich Taste of Friendship
An extra helping

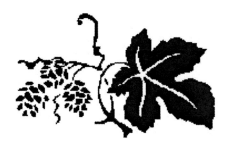

"When I find myself fading, I close my eyes and realize my friends are my energy."
-Anonymous

"The road to a friend's house is never long."
-Danish proverb

"Friendship is the hardest thing in the world to explain. It's not something you learn in school. But if you haven't learned the meaning of friendship, you really haven't learned anything."
-Muhammad Ali

"A friendship can weather most things and thrive in thin soil; but it needs a little mulch of letters and phone calls and small, silly presents every so often – just to save it from drying out completely."
-Pam Brown

"Friends are treasures."
-Horace Bruns

"An insincere and evil friend is more to be feared than a wild beast; a wild beast may wound your body, but an evil friend will wound your mind."
-Buddha

"The only way to have a friend is to be one."
-Ralph Waldo Emerson

"He who has a thousand friends
Has not a friend to spare,
While he who has one enemy
Shall meet him everywhere."
-Ralph Waldo Emerson

"A friend is one who knows you
and loves you just the same."
-Elbert Hubbard

"The real test of friendship is: can you literally do
nothing with the other person? Can you
enjoy those moments of
life that are utterly simple?"
-Eugene Kennedy

"We call that person who has lost his father, an orphan;
and a widower that man who has lost his wife. But
that man who has known the immense unhappiness of
losing a friend, by what name do we call him?
Here every language is silent
and holds its peace in impotence."
-Joseph Roux

"Be courteous to all, but intimate with few, and let those
few be well tried before you give them your confidence.
True friendship is a plant of slow grow, and must
undergo and withstand the shocks of adversity before
it is entitled to the appellation."
-George Washington

Creativity, Persistence, Courage, and Imagination
Soul Food

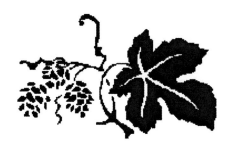

"Time is money."
-Benjamin Franklin, *Advice to a Young Tradesman*

"The way to get things done is not to mind who gets the credit for doing them."
-Benjamin Jowett

"Joy is but the sign that creative emotion is fulfilling its purpose."
-Charles Du Bos, *What Is Literature?*

"Creative minds have always been known to survive any kind of bad training."
-Anna Freud

"The deepest experience of the creator is feminine, for it is experience of receiving and bearing."
-Rainer Maria Rilke, *Letters of Rainer Maria Rilke*

"The very essence of the creative is its novelty, and hence we have no standard by which to judge it."
-Carl R. Rogers, *On Becoming a Person*

"Any activity becomes creative when the doer cares about doing it right, or doing it better."
-John Updike

"There are no shortcuts to any place worth going."
-Anonymous

"It's the constant and determined effort that breaks down resistance, sweeps away all obstacles."
-Claude M. Bristol

"It is no use saying, 'We are doing our best.' You have got to succeed in doing what is necessary."
-Sir Winston Churchill

"Efficiency is intelligent laziness."
-David Dunham

We aim above the mark to hit the mark."
-Ralph Waldo Emerson

"You get the best out of others when
you give the best of yourself."
-Harry Firestone

"One that would have the fruit must climb the tree."
-Thomas Fuller

"Knowing is not enough; we must apply.
Willing is not enough; we must do."
-Johann von Goethe

"The harder you work, the luckier you get."
-McAlexander

"It's always too early to quit."
-Norman Vincent Peale

"Slump, and the world slumps with you.
Push, and you push alone."
-Laurence J. Peter

"Even if you are on the right track, you'll
get run over if you just sit there."
-Will Rogers

"Do what you can, with what you have, where you are."
-Theodore Roosevelt

"To do two things at once is to do neither."
-Publilius Syrus

"Reality can be beaten with enough imagination."
-Anonymous

"There is a boundary to men's passions when they act
from feelings; but none when they are under
the influence of imagination."
-Edmund Burke

"Live out of your imagination, not your history."
-Stephen Covey

"Imagination is more important than knowledge.
Knowledge is limited. Imagination encircles the world."
-Albert Einstein

"To imagine is everything, to know is nothing at all."
-Anatole France, The Crime of Sylvester Bernard, 1881

"Imagination is the only weapon
in the war against reality."
-Jules de Gautier

"Some men see things as they are and ask, 'why?' I
dream things that never were and ask, 'why not?'"
* This quote is a paraphrase from a similar quote by G. B. Shaw.
-Robert Francis Kennedy

"Imagination grows by exercise, and contrary to
common belief, is more powerful in the
mature than in the young."
-W. Somerset Maugham

"You see things as they are and ask, 'Why?' I dream
things as they never were and ask, 'Why not?'"
-George Bernard Shaw

"Consistency is the last resort of the unimaginative."
-Oscar Wilde

"I am imagination. I can see what the eyes cannot see. I
can hear what the ears cannot hear. I can feel
what the heart cannot feel."
-Peter Nivio Zarlenga

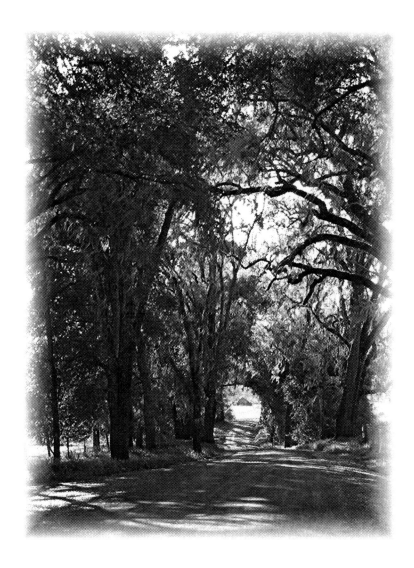

Greatness
Crème de la Crème

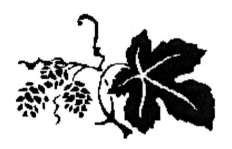

"They're only truly great who are truly good."
-George Chapman

"The price of greatness is responsibility."
-Sir Winston Churchill

"Nothing great was ever achieved without enthusiasm."
-Ralph Waldo Emerson

"Nothing great in the world has ever been
accomplished without passion."
-G. W. F. Hegel

"Great deeds are usually wrought at great risks."
-Herodotus

"The greatest thing a man can do in this world is to
make the most possible out of the stuff that has been
given him. This is success, and there is no other."
-Orison Swett Marden

"Don't dwell on reality; it will only
keep you from greatness."
-Rev. Randall R. McBride, Jr.

"There are countless ways of achieving greatness, but
any road to achieving one's maximum potential must
be built on a bedrock of respect for the
individual, a commitment to excellence,
and a rejection of mediocrity."
-Buck Rodgers

"Be not afraid of greatness: some are born great, some
achieve greatness, and some have greatness
thrust upon them."
-William Shakespeare

"To endure is greater than to dare; to tire out hostile
fortune; to be daunted by no difficulty; to keep heart
when all have lost it -- who can say
this is not greatness?"
-William Makepeace Thackeray

"There are no great things, only small things
with great love. Happy are those."
-Mother Theresa

Virtue, Strength, and Patience
Key Ingredients of Life

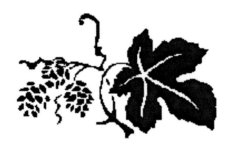

"Nothing in this world can take the place of persistence. Talent will not; nothing is more common than unsuccessful people with talent. Genius will not; unrewarded genius is almost a proverb. Education will not; the world is full of educated derelicts. Persistence and determination alone are omnipotent. The slogan 'press on' has solved and always will solve the problems of the human race."
-Calvin Coolidge

"Success seems to be largely a matter of hanging on after others have let go."
-William Feather

"Diamonds are nothing more than chunks of coal that stuck to their jobs."
-Malcolm Stevenson Forbes

"When you get to the end of your rope, tie a knot and hang on."
-Franklin D. Roosevelt

"Fall seven times, stand up eight."
-Japanese Proverb

"Our greatest glory is not in ever falling, but in rising every time we fall."
-Confucius

"It is said an eastern monarch once charged his wise men to invent a sentence, to be ever in view, and which should be true and appropriate in all times and situations. They presented him with the words, **'And this, too, shall pass away.'** How much it expresses! How chastening in the hour of pride! How consoling in the depths of affliction!
-Abraham Lincoln

"I learned that it is the weak who are cruel, and that gentleness is to be expected only from the strong."
-Leo Rosten

"Nothing is so strong as gentleness and nothing is so gentle as real strength."
-Ralph W. Sockman

"We deceive ourselves when we fancy that only weakness needs support. Strength needs it far more."
-Madame Swetchine, The Writings of Madame Swetchine

"The soul that is within me no man can degrade."
-Frederick Douglas

"Where talent is a dwarf, self-esteem is a giant."
-J. Petit-Senn, Conceits and Caprices

"This above all; to thine own self be true."
-William Shakespeare

"Virtue is not the absence of vices or the avoidance of moral dangers; virtue is a vivid and separate thing, like pain or a particular smell."
-G. K. Chesterton, Tremendous Trifles

"Modesty is a vastly overrated virtue."
-John Kenneth Galbraith

"Virtue herself is her own fairest reward."
-Silius Italicus, Punica

"Nature does not loathe virtue: it is unaware of its existence."
-Françoise Mallet-Joris, A Letter to Myself

"Man cannot be uplifted; he must be seduced into virtue."
-Don Marquis, The Almost Perfect State

"And be on thy guard against the good and the just! They would fain crucify those who devise their own virtue -- they hate the lonesome ones."
-Friedrich Nietzsche, Thus Spake Zarathustra

"Speak softly and carry a big stick; you will go far."
-Theodore Roosevelt, 1901

"The glory that goes with wealth is fleeting and fragile;
virtue is a possession glorious and eternal."
-Sallust

"It is a revenge the devil sometimes takes upon the
virtuous, that he entraps them by the force of the very
passion they have suppressed and
think themselves superior to."
-George Santayana, The Letters of George Santayana

"Honest disagreement is often a good sign of progress."
-Mahatma Gandhi

"Yesterday we obeyed kings and bent our necks before
emperors. But today we kneel only to truth,
follow only beauty, and obey only love."
-Kahlil Gibran, "Children of Gods, Scions of Apes"

"Progress lies not in enhancing what is, but
in advancing toward what will be."
-Kahlil Gibran, "A Handful of Sand on the Shore"

"The universe is full of magical things, patiently
waiting for our wits to grow sharper."
-Eden Phillpotts

"There are many ways of going forward,
but only one way of standing still."
-Franklin D. Roosevelt

"Progress, far from consisting in change, depends on
retentiveness. Those who cannot remember the
past are condemned to repeat it."
-George Santayana

"Reasonable people adapt themselves to the world.
Unreasonable people attempt to adapt the world
to themselves. All progress, therefore, depends on
unreasonable people."
-George Bernard Shaw

"Our patience will achieve more than our force."
-Edmund Burke, *Reflections on the Revolution in France, 1790*

"Beware the fury of a patient man."
-John Dryden, *Absalom and Achitophel, 1681*

"All commend patience, but none can endure to suffer."
-Thomas Fuller, *Gnomologia, 1732*

"Let him that hath no power of patience retire within
himself, though even there he will
have to put up with himself."
-Baltasar Gracian, *The Art of Worldy Wisdom, 1647*

"Patience makes lighter
What sorrow may not heal."
-Horace, *Odes, 15*

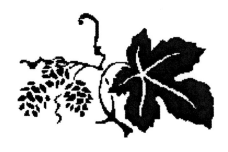

Truth and Wealth
A blend of ingredients

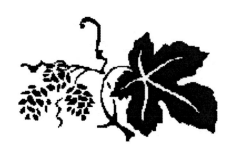

"As scarce as truth is, the supply has always
been in excess of the demand."
-Josh Billings

"When I tell the truth, it is not for the sake of
convincing those who do not know it, but for the sake
of defending those that do."
-William Blake

"The object of the superior man is truth."
-Confucius

"It is an old maxim of mine that when you have excluded
the impossible, whatever remains, however
improbable, must be the truth."
-Conan Doyle, The Adventures of Sherlock Holmes,
"The Beryl Coronet"

"Once the toothpaste is out of the tube,
it's hard to get it back in!"
-H.R. Haldeman

"Pretty much all the honest truth-telling there is in
the world is done by children."
-Oliver Wendell Holmes

"No one is entitled to the truth."
-E. Howard Hunt

"You shall know the truth, and the truth
shall make you mad."
-Aldous Huxley

"It is error alone which needs the support of government.
Truth can stand by itself."
-Thomas Jefferson

"It is always the best policy to speak the truth, unless,
of course, you are an exceptionally good liar."
-Jerome K. Jerome

"A lie told often enough becomes truth."
-Lenin (Vladimir Ulyanov)

"It is hard to believe that a man is telling the truth when
you know that you would lie if you were in his place."
-H. L. Mencken

"All great truths begin as blasphemies."
-George Bernard Shaw

"Be true to your work, your word, and your friend."
-Henry David Thoreau

"If you tell the truth, you don't
have to remember anything."
-Mark Twain

"The pure and simple truth is rarely pure
and never simple."
-Oscar Wilde

"The real measure of your wealth is how much you'd be
worth if you lost all your money."
-Anonymous

"The world at large does not judge us by who we are and
what we know; it judges us by what we have."
-Joyce Brothers

"My riches consist not in the extent of my possessions,
but in the fewness of my wants."
-J. Brotherton

"There's no reason to be the richest man in the cemetery.
You can't do any business from there."
-Colonel Sanders

"Real riches are the riches possessed inside."
-B. C. Forbes

"If you can count your money, you don't
have a billion dollars."
-J. Paul Getty

"Would that I were a dry well, and that the people tossed
stones into me, for that would be easier than to be a
spring of flowing water that the thirsty
pass by, and from which they avoid drinking."
-Kahlil Gibran, "My Soul Is Heavy Laden with its Fruits"

"Poverty is a veil that obscures the face of greatness. An
appeal is a mask covering the face of tribulation."
-Kahlil Gibran, "A Handful of Sand on the Shore"

"The trouble with being poor is that
it takes up all your time."
-Willem de Kooning

"The rich are different from you and me
because they have more credit."
-John Leonard

"I don't know much about being a millionaire,
but I'll bet I'd be darling at it."
-Dorothy Parker

"I'd like to live as a poor man with lots of money."
-Pablo Picasso

"Wealth is the product of man's capacity to think."
-Ayn Rand

"What difference does it make how much you have?
What you do not have amounts to much more."
-Seneca

"A man is rich in proportion to the number of
things he can let alone."
-Henry David Thoreau, Walden

"A fool and his money are soon parted."
-Thomas Tusser, Five Hundred Points of Good Husbandry

"The more money an American accumulates,
the less interesting he becomes."
-Gore Vidal

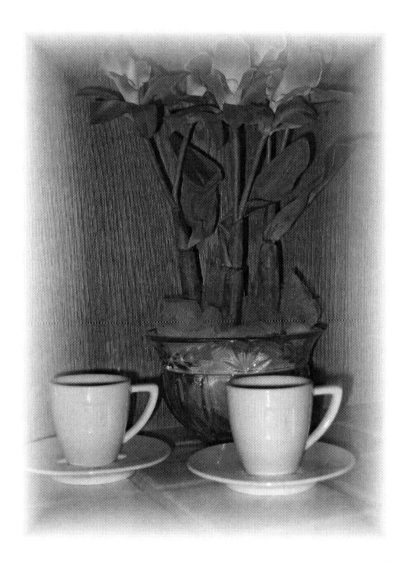

Loyalty, Opportunity, and Success
The Spice of Life

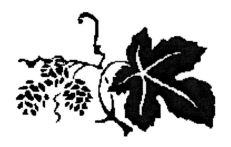

"Loyalty is still the same,
Whether it win or lose the game;
True as a dial to the sun,
Although it be not shined upon."
-Samuel Butler, Hudibras, 1663

"If I had to choose between betraying my country and
betraying my friend, I hope I should have the
guts to betray my country."
-E. M. Forster, Two Cheers for Democracy

"Opportunity may knock only once,
but temptation leans on the doorbell."
-Anonymous

"Many an opportunity is lost because a man
is out looking for four-leaf clovers."
-Anonymous

"The golden opportunity you are seeking is in yourself.
It is not in your environment; it is
not in luck or chance, or the
help of others; it is in yourself alone."
-Orison Swett Marden

"Most successful men have not achieved their
distinction by having some new talent or opportunity
presented to them. They have developed the
opportunity that was at hand."
-Bruce Marton

"Fortune knocks but once, but misfortune
has much more patience."
-Laurence J. Peter

"We are confronted with insurmountable opportunities."
-Pogo

"The doors we open and close each
day decide the lives we live."
-Flora Whittemore

"A man should not strive to eliminate his complexes but
to get into accord with them: they are legitimately
what directs his conduct in the world."
-Sigmund Freud

"Man's main task in life is to give birth to himself,
to become what he potentially is.
The most important product
of his effort is his own personality."
-Erich Fromm, Man for Himself

"It is by no means certain that our individual
personality is the single inhabitant of these our
corporeal frames... We all do things both awake and
asleep which surprise us. Perhaps
we have cotenants in this house we live in."
-Oliver Wendell Holmes, *The Guardian Angel*

"A good head and a good heart are always
a formidable combination."
-Nelson Mandela

"Personality is born out of pain.
It is the fire shut up in the flint."
-J. B. Yeats, *Letters to His Son, W. B. Yeats and Others*

"Success always occurs in private,
and failure in full view."
-Anonymous

"Eighty percent of success is showing up."
-Woody Allen

"If you find it in your heart to care for somebody
else you will have succeeded."
-Maya Angelou

"For many are called, but few are chosen."
-Matthew 22:14

"They never fail who die in a great cause."
-George Gordon Byron

"The important thing to recognize is that it takes a team, and the team ought to get credit for the wins and the losses. Successes have many fathers, failures have none."
-Philip Caldwell

"I don't know the key to success, but the key to failure is to try to please everyone."
-Bill Cosby

"The thermometer of success is merely the jealousy of the malcontents."
-Salvador Dali

"Defeat never comes to any man until he admits it."
-Josephus Daniels

"Try not to become a man of success, but rather
try to become a man of value."
-Albert Einstein

"To laugh often and much; to win the respect of
intelligent people and the affection of children; to
earn the appreciation of honest critics and endure
the betrayal of false friends; to appreciate beauty,
to find the best in others; to leave the world a little
better; whether by a healthy child, a garden patch or
a redeemed social condition; to know even one life
has breathed easier because you have lived. This is the
meaning of success."
-Ralph Waldo Emerson

"But man is not made for defeat. A man can
be destroyed but not defeated."
-Ernest Hemingway

"The majority of men meet with failure because of their
lack of persistence in creating new plans to
take the place of those which fail."
-Napoleon Hill

"Only those who dare to fail greatly can
ever achieve greatly."
-Robert Francis Kennedy

"It's not failure, but low aim is crime."
-Lowell

"Success is that old ABC -- ability, breaks, and courage."
-Charles Luckman

"No man succeeds without a good woman behind him. Wife or mother, if it is both, he is twice blessed indeed."
-Harold MacMillan, 1963

"You may be disappointed if you fail, but you are doomed if you don't try."
-Beverly Sills

"The only time you don't fail is the last time you try anything -- and it works."
-William Strong

"Men are born to succeed, not to fail."
-Henry David Thoreau

"Sometimes I worry about being a success in a mediocre world."
-Lily Tomlin

59

"Success in almost any field depends more on energy and drive than it does on intelligence. This explains why we have so many stupid leaders."
-Sloan Wilson

"Nothing recedes like success."
-Walter Winchell

"Defeat is not the worst of failures.
Not to have tried is the true failure."
-George E. Woodberry

"What you do speaks so loudly that
I cannot hear what you say."
-Ralph Waldo Emerson

"To avoid criticism, do nothing, say nothing,
and be nothing."
-Elbert Hubbard

"Never believe that a few caring people can't change the world. For, indeed, that's all who ever have."
-Margaret Mead

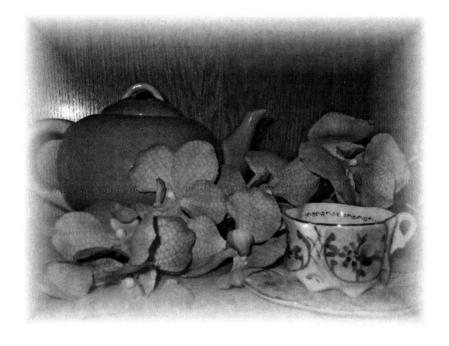

<u>Happiness</u>
The icing on the cake

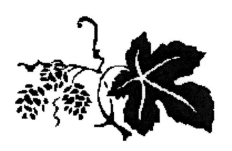

"Happiness is a choice that requires effort at times."
-Anonymous

"Be happy while you're living, for
you're a long time dead."
-Scottish Proverb

"Most people would rather be certain they're
miserable, than risk being happy."
-Robert Anthony

"...happiness is the highest good, being a realization
and perfect practice of virtue, which some can attain,
while others have little or none of it..."
-Aristotle

"People take different roads seeking fulfillment and
happiness. Just because they're not on your road doesn't
mean they've gotten lost."
-H. Jackson Brown, Jr.

"To live a pure unselfish life, one must count nothing
as one's own in the midst of abundance."
-Buddha

"Action may not always bring happiness; but
there is no happiness without action."
-Benjamin Disraeli

"The Constitution only gives people the right to pursue
happiness. You have to catch it yourself."
-Ben Franklin

"He is happiest, be he king or peasant,
who finds peace in his home."
-Johann von Goethe

"Happiness is not a destination. It is a method of life."
-Burton Hills

"When one door of happiness closes, another opens; but
often we look so long at the closed
door that we do not see the
one which has opened for us."
-Helen Keller

"I have no money, no resources, no hopes.
I am the happiest man alive."
-Henry Miller

"Nobody really cares if you're miserable,
so you might as well be happy."
-Cynthia Nelms

"Good humor is one of the best articles of
dress one can wear in society."
-William Makepeace Thackeray

"The best way to cheer yourself up is to
try to cheer somebody else up."
-Mark Twain

"Some cause happiness wherever they
go; others whenever they go."
-Oscar Wilde

"Those who bring sunshine to the lives of others
cannot keep it from themselves."
-James Barrie

"If you can't return a favor, pass it on."
-Louise Brown

"Darkness cannot drive out darkness; only
light can do that. Hate cannot drive out hate;
only love can do that."
-Martin Luther King, Jr.

"We must use time wisely and forever realize that the
time is always ripe to do right."
-Nelson Mendela

"After the verb 'to Love,' 'to Help' is the most
beautiful verb in the world."
-Bertha von Suttner

"No pessimist ever discovered the secrets of stars, or
sailed to an uncharted land, or opened a new
heaven to the human spirit."
- Helen Keller

Decision and Choice
With or without nuts

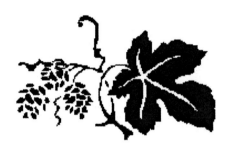

"We can try to avoid making choices by doing nothing, but even that is a decision."
-Gary Collins

"Most of the things we decide are not what we know to be the best. We say yes, merely because we are driven into a corner and must say something."
-Frank Crane, Essays

"When making a decision of minor importance, I have always found it advantageous to consider all the pros and cons. In vital matters, however, such as the choice of a mate or a profession, the decision should come from the unconscious, from somewhere within ourselves. In the important decisions of personal life, we should be governed, I think, by the deep inner needs of our nature."
-Sigmund Freud

"If one does not know to which port one is sailing, no wind is favorable."
-Seneca

"Choice has always been a privilege of those who could afford to pay for it."
-Ellen Frankfort

"We choose our joys and sorrows long
before we experience them."
-Kahlil Gibran, *Sand and Foam*

"Would ye both eat your cake and have your cake?"
This is commonly misquoted as
"You can't have your cake and eat it, too."
-John Heywood, *John Heywood's Proverbs, 1546*

"I think there is choice possible to us at any moment,
as long as we live. But there is no sacrifice. There is a
choice, and the rest falls away. Second choice does not
exist. Beware of those who talk about sacrifice."
-Muriel Rukeyser, *The Life of Poetry*

"Everybody wants to be somebody;
nobody wants to grow."
-Johann von Goethe

"The rung of a ladder was never meant to rest upon, but
only to hold a man's foot long enough to enable
him to put the other somewhat higher."
-Thomas Henry Huxley, *Life and Letters of Thomas Huxley*

"I know that every good and excellent thing in the
world stands moment by moment on the razor-edge of
danger and must be fought for..."
-Thornton Wilder

"I do not think much of a man who is not
wiser today than he was yesterday."
-Abraham Lincoln

"There was that law of life, so cruel and so just, that one
must grow or else pay more for remaining the same."
-Norman Mailer, The Deer Park

"When we blindly adopt a religion, a political system,
a literary dogma, we become automatons.
We cease to grow."
-Anaïs Nin, The Diaries of Anaïs Nin

"Indecision is like a stepchild: if he does not wash his
hands, he is called dirty, if he does, he is wasting water."
-African Proverb

"The whole world steps aside for the man
who knows where he is going."
-Anonymous

"One's mind has a way of making itself up in the
background, and it suddenly becomes
clear what one means to do."
-A. C. Benson

"When you realize the value of all life, you dwell less
on what is past and concentrate more on the
preservation of the future."
- Dian Fossey

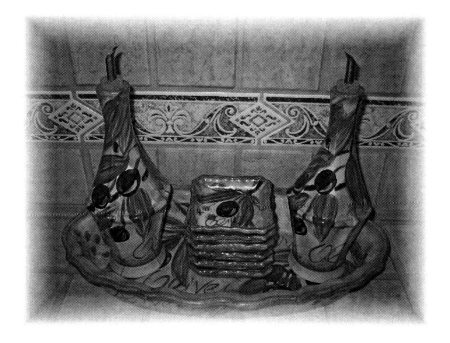

Honesty, Destiny, and Knowledge
The aroma of positive thinking

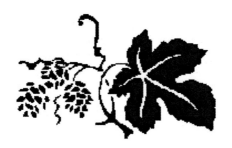

"Oh, what a tangled web we weave,
When first we practice to deceive!"
-Sir Walter Scott, Marmion

"No legacy is so rich as honesty."
-William Shakespeare

"Each time you are honest and conduct yourself with
honesty, a success force will drive you toward greater
success. Each time you lie, even with a little
white lie, there are strong forces
pushing you toward failure."
-Joseph Sugarman

"Only the spoon knows what is stirring in the pot."
-Sicilian Proverb

"Real knowledge is to know the extent
of one's ignorance."
-Confucius

"Knowledge cultivates your seeds
and does not sow in you seeds."
-Kahlil Gibran, "A Handful of Sand on the Shore"

"Knowledge is of two kinds. We know a subject
ourselves, or we know where we can find
information upon it."
-Samuel Johnson

"There is much pleasure not be gained
from useless knowledge."
-Bertrand Russell

"Knowledge of the self is the mother of all knowledge.
So it is incumbent on me to know my self, to know it
completely, to know its minutiae, its characteristics,
its subtleties, and its very atoms."
-Kahlil Gibran, "The Philosophy of Logic"

"The unexamined life is not worth living."
-Socrates

"One thing you can't recycle is wasted time."
-Anonymous

"Obstacles are those frightful things you see when
you take your eyes off your goal."
-Henry Ford

"This one step – choosing a goal and sticking
to it – changes everything."
-Scott Reed

"The indispensable first step to getting
the things you want out of life is this:
decide what you want."
-Ben Stein

"Not all who wander are lost."
-J. R. R. Tolkien

"Destiny is not a matter of chance, it is a matter of
choice; it is not a thing to be waited for, it is
a thing to be achieved."
-William Jennings Bryan

"I have always believed that all things depended upon
fortune, and nothing upon ourselves."
-George Gordon Byron

"It is to be remarked that a good many people are born
curiously unfitted for the fate waiting
them on this earth."
-Joseph Conrad, Chance

"Lots of folks confuse bad management with destiny."
-Kim Hubbard

"And when man faces destiny, destiny
ends and man comes into his own."
-André Malraux, The Voices of Silence

"Every man has his own destiny: the only imperative is
to follow it, to accept it, no matter where it leads him."
-Henry Miller, The Wisdom of the Heart

"It is not in the stars to hold our
destiny but in ourselves."
-William Shakespeare

Generosity and Excellence

All natural ingredients

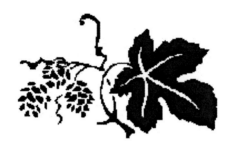

"No one is so generous as he who has nothing to give."
-French Proverb

"Generosity is not giving me that which I need more
than you do, but it is giving me that
which you need more than I do."
-Kahlil Gibran, Sand and Foam

"The return we reap from generous
actions is not always evident."
-Francesco Guicciardini, Counsels and Reflections

"The true meaning of life is to plant trees, under
whose shade you do not expect to sit."
-Nelson Henderson

"I am convinced that the majority of people would be
generous from selfish motives,
if they had the opportunity."
-Charles Dudley Warner, My Summer in a Garden

"Do all the good you can, by all the means you can, in
all the ways you can, in all the places you can, at all
the times you can, to all the people you can,
as long as ever you can."
-John Wesley

"Good, better, best; never let it rest till your good is better and your better is best."
-Anonymous

"We are what we repeatedly do. Excellence, then, is not an act, but a habit."
-Aristotle

"Hold yourself responsible for a higher standard than anybody expects of you. Never excuse yourself."
-Henry Ward Beecher

"Before the gates of excellence the high gods have placed sweat; long is the road thereto and rough and steep at first; but when the heights are reached, then there is ease, though grievously hard in the winning."
-Hesiod, Works and Days

"Real excellence and humility are not incompatible one with the other, on the contrary they are twin sisters."
-Jean Baptiste Lacordaire, Letters to Young Men

"Success will not lower its standard to us.
We must raise our standard to success."
-Rev. Randall R. McBride, Jr.

"Excellence is not a singular act, but a habit.
You are what you repeatedly do."
* This quotation is a paraphrase of a much older quote by Aristotle
-Shaquille O'Neal

"There ought to be so many who are excellent,
there are so few."
-Janet Erskine Stuart

"God is in the details."
-Mies van der Rohe, "New York Times", August 19, 1969

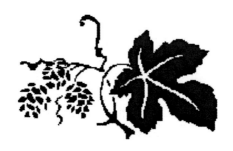

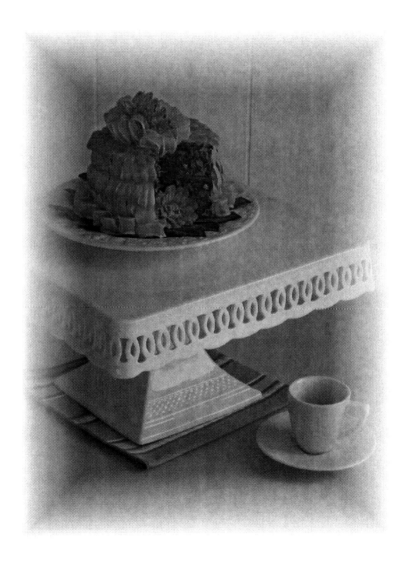

<u>Laughter</u>
Dessert without the calories

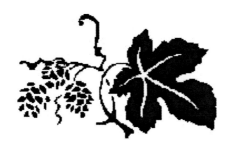

"Men show their character in nothing more clearly
than by what they find laughable."
-Anonymous

"Nobody ever died of laughter."
-Max Beerbohm

"Laughter is the shortest distance between two people."
-Victor Borge

"The most wasted day of all is that during
which we have not laughed."
-Sebastian R. N. Chamfort

"Laughter is nothing else but a sudden glory arising
from some sudden conception of some eminency
in ourselves, by comparison with the infirmity
of others, or with our own formerly."
-Thomas Hobbes

"If you don't learn to laugh at troubles, you won't have anything to laugh at when you grow old."
-Edward W. Howe

"Perhaps I know why it is man alone who laughs: He alone suffers so deeply that he had to invent laughter."
-Friedrich Nietzsche

"Life does not cease to be funny when people die any more than it ceases to be serious when people laugh."
-George Bernard Shaw

"The human race has one really effective weapon, and that is laughter."
-Mark Twain

"Humor is an affirmation of man's dignity, a declaration of man's superiority to all that befalls him."
-Romain Cary

"Humor is not a postscript or an incidental afterthought; it is a serious and weighty part of the world's economy. One feels increasingly the height of the faculty in which it arises, the nobility of things associated with it, and
the greatness of services it renders."
-Oscar W. Firkins, Oscar Firkins: Memoirs and Letters

"Humor is perhaps a sense of intellectual perspective: an awareness that some things are really important, others not; and that the two kinds are most oddly jumbled in everyday affairs."
-Christopher Morley, Inward Ho

"Humor distorts nothing, and only false gods are laughed off their earthly pedestals."
-Agnes Repplier, Points of View

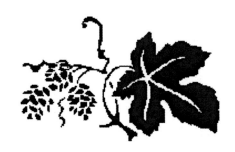

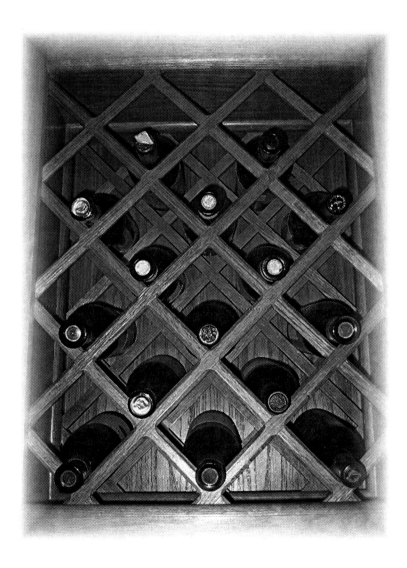

Forgiveness
Diluting the intensity

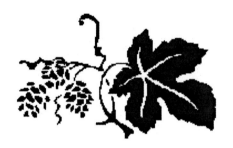

"It is easier to forgive an enemy than to forgive a friend."
-William Blake, Jerusalem, 1820

"Reason to rule but mercy to forgive:
The first is the law, the last prerogative."
-John Dryden, "The Hind and the Panther", 1687

"Forgiveness is the answer to the child's dream of a
miracle by which what is broken
is made whole again, what
is soiled is made clean again."
-Dag Hammarskjöld, Markings, 1964

"The ineffable joy of forgiving and being forgiven
forms an ecstasy that might well arouse
the envy of the gods."
-Elbert Hubbard, The Note Book, 1927

"Forgive your enemies, but never forget their names."
-John Fitzgerald Kennedy

"If there is something to pardon in everything,
there is also something to condemn."
-Friedrich Nietzsche, The Will to Power, 1888

"To err is human; to forgive, divine."
-Alexander Pope, "An Essay on Criticism"

"What power has love but forgiveness?
In other words
by its intervention
what has been done
can be undone.
What good is it otherwise?"
-William Carlos Williams, Pictures from Brueghel,
1962

<u>Change</u>
Expanding your palate

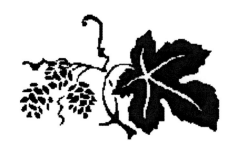

"To change and to change for the better
re two different things."
-German proverb

"If you don't like something, change it. If you can't
change it, change your attitude. Don't complain."
-Maya Angelou

"Any change, even a change for the better, is always
accompanied by drawbacks and discomforts."
-Arnold Bennett, "The Arnold Bennett Calendar"

"Only the wisest and stupidest of men never change."
-Confucius

"Without change, something sleeps inside us, and
seldom awakens. The sleeper must awaken."
-Frank Herbert

"We live in a moment of history
where change is so speeded
up that we begin to see the present only
when it is already disappearing."
-R. D. Laing, The Politics of Experience

"None of us knows what the next change is going to be,
what unexpected opportunity is just around the corner,
waiting a few months or a few years to
change all the tenor of our lives."
-Kathleen Norris, Hands Full of Living

"If we don't change, we don't grow. If we
don't grow, we aren't really living."
-Gail Sheehy

"We are chameleons, and our partialities and
prejudices change place with an easy
and blessed facility, and we are
soon wanted to the change and happy in it."
-Mark Twain, Mark Twain at Your Fingertips

"He is able who thinks he is able."
-Buddha

"A man must not deny his manifest abilities,
for that is to evade his obligations."
-William Feather, The Treasure of Franchard

"You must be the change you wish to see in the world."
-Mahatma Gandhi

"Great ability develops and reveals itself
increasingly with every new assignment."
-Baltasar Gracian, The Oracle

"A person who aims at nothing is sure to hit it."
-Anonymous

"We are told never to cross a bridge until we come to it,
but this world is owned by men
who have 'crossed bridges' in their
imagination far ahead of the crowd"
-Anonymous

"No bird soars too high if he soars with his own wings."
-William Blake

"Shoot for the moon. Even if you miss,
you'll land among the stars."
-Les Brown

"You can't build a reputation on
what you're going to do."
-Henry Ford

"To accomplish great things, we must not only act, but
also dream; not only plan, but also believe."
-Anatole France

"The best way out is always through."
-Robert Frost

"Don't be afraid to take a big step. You can't
cross a chasm in two small jumps."
-David Lloyd George

"Advance, and never halt, for advancing is perfection.
Advance and do not fear the thorns in the path,
for they draw only corrupt blood."
-Kahlil Gibran, "The Visit of Wisdom"

"Hold fast to dreams, for if dreams die, life is a
broken winged bird that cannot fly."
-Langston Hughes

"An ounce of hypocrisy is worth a pound of ambition."
-Michael Korda

"The entrepreneur is essentially a visualizer and an
actualizer... He can visualize something,
and when he visualizes it he sees exactly
how to make it happen."
-Robert L. Schwartz

"The roots of true achievement lie in the will
to become the best that you can become."
-Harold Taylor

"Keep away from people who try to belittle your
ambitions. Small people always do that,
but the really great make
you feel that you, too, can become great."
-Mark Twain

"If you can imagine it,
You can achieve it.
If you can dream it,
You can become it."
-William Arthur Ward

"I'd rather be a could-be if I cannot be an are;
because a could-be is a maybe who is
reaching for a star. I'd rather be a
has-been than a might-have-been, by far; for a might
have-been has never been, but a has was once an are."
-Milton Berle

"In the depths of winter I finally learned there
was in me an invincible summer."
-Albert Camus

"Zeal is a volcano, the peak of which the grass of
indecisiveness does not grow."
-Kahlil Gibran, "A Handful of Sand on the Shore"

"The tears that you spill, the sorrowful, are sweeter than
the laughter of snobs and the guffaws of scoffers."
-Kahlil Gibran, "A Handful of Sand on the Shore"

"An inexhaustible good nature is one of the most
precious gifts of heaven, spreading itself like oil over
the troubled sea of thought, and keeping the mind
smooth and equable in the roughest weather."
-Washington Irving

"No pessimist ever discovered the secret of the stars, or
sailed to an uncharted land, or opened a new
doorway for the human spirit."
-Helen Keller

"A will finds a way."
-Orison Swett Marden

"God grant me the serenity to accept the things I cannot change, the courage to change the things I can, and the wisdom to know the difference."
-Reinhold Niebuhr

"She would rather light candles than curse the darkness and her glow has warmed the world."
-Adlai Stevenson,
Eulogy of Eleanor Roosevelt, November 7, 1962

"Every exit is an entry somewhere."
-Tom Stoppard

"The cynic knows the price of everything and the value of nothing."
-Oscar Wilde, "Lady Windemere's Fan"

"You can complain because roses have thorns, or you can rejoice because thorns have roses."
-Ziggy

"Work joyfully and peacefully, knowing that right thoughts and right efforts inevitably bring about right results."
-James Allen

"The best-laid schemes o' mice an 'men
gang aft agley."
-Robert Burns, "To A Mouse"

"Image creates desire. You will what you imagine."
-J. G. Gallimore

"'He means well' is useless unless he does well."
-Plautus

"Nothing happens by itself... it all will come your way,
once you understand that you have to make it come
your way, by your own exertions."
-Ben Stein

"No one is listening until you make a mistake."
-Anonymous

"Every man has his follies – and often they are
the most interesting thing he has got."
-Josh Billings

"There are no mistakes, no coincidences. All events
are blessings given to us to learn from."
-Elizabeth Kubler-Ross

"The only real mistake is the one from
which we learn nothing."
-John Powell

"When they discover the center of the universe, a lot of
people will be disappointed to discover they are not it."
-Bernard Bailey

"Never look down on anybody unless
you are helping him up."
-Jesse Jackson

"Many a man is praised for his reserve and so-called
shyness when he is simply too proud to
risk making a fool of himself."
-J. B. Priestley, All About Ourselves and Other Essays

"There is no such thing as a long piece of work,
except one that you dare not start."
-Charles Baudelaire, Intimate Journals

"'We must do something' is the unanimous refrain.
'You begin' is the deadening refrain."
-Walter Dwight, The Saving Sense

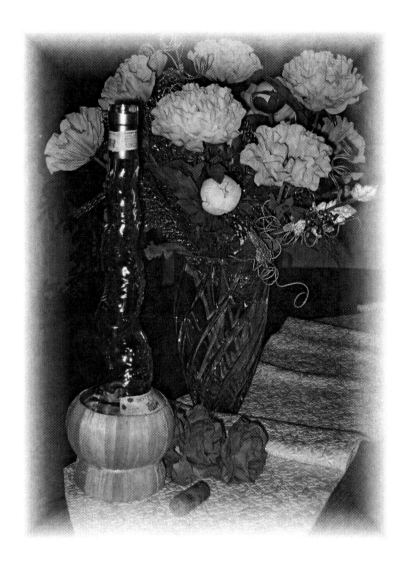

Time
Just in Thyme – Baked to Perfection

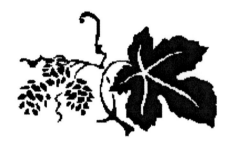

"Time goes by so fast, people go in and out of your life.
You must never miss the opportunity to tell these
people how much they mean to you."
-"Cheers"

"Let him who would enjoy a good future
waste none of his present."
-Roger Babson

"You can never plan the future by the past."
-Edmund Burke

"You may delay, but time will not."
-Benjamin Franklin

"Time has been transformed, and we have changed; it
has advanced and set us in motion; it has unveiled its
face, inspiring us with bewilderment and exhilaration."
-Kahlil Gibran, "Children of Gods, Scions of Apes"

"Until you value yourself, you won't value your time.
Until you value your time, you will not
do anything with it."
-M Scott Peck

"Time is the fire in which we burn."
-Gene Roddenberry

"Everything happens to everybody sooner or
later if there is time enough."
-George Bernard Shaw

"The trouble with our times is that the
future is not what it used to be."
-Paul Valery

"We never know the worth of water 'til the well is dry."
-English Proverb

"Not everything that can be counted counts, and not
everything that counts can be counted."
-Albert Einstein

"One should never criticize his own work except in a
fresh and hopeful mood. The self-criticism
of a tired mind is suicide."
-Charles Horton Cooley, Life and the Student

Words of Measure
Getting your fill of snacks

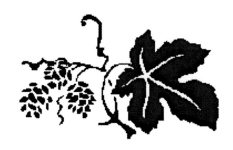

"Honest criticism is hard to take,
particularly from a relative,
a friend, an acquaintance or a stranger."
-Franklin Jones

"It is salutary to train oneself to be no more
affected by censure than by praise."
-W. Somerset Maugham, The Summing Up

"Our character is what we do when
we think no one is looking."
-H. Jackson Brown, Jr.

"To measure the man, measure his heart."
-Malcolm Stevenson Forbes

"The true test of character is not how much we know
how to do, but how we behave when we
don't know what to do."
-John Holt

"Many a man's reputation would not know his
character if they met on the street."
-Elbert Hubbard

"Character cannot be developed in ease and quiet. Only
through experience of trial and suffering can the soul be
strengthened, ambition inspired, and success achieved."
-Helen Keller

"A loving person lives in a loving world. A hostile person lives in a hostile world.
Everyone you meet is your mirror."
-Ken Keys

"The ultimate measure of a man is not where he stands in moments of comfort, but where he stands at times of challenge and controversy."
-Martin Luther King, Jr.

"Nearly all men can stand adversity, but if you want to test a man's character, give him power."
-Abraham Lincoln

"Bluntness is a virtue."
-Allison Ling

"The measure of a man's real character is what he would do if he knew he would never be found out."
-Thomas B. Macaulay

"It's good to shut up sometimes."
-Marcel Marceau

"When you choose your friends, don't be short-
changed by choosing personality over character."
-W. Somerset Maugham

"Make your life a mission – not an intermission."
-Arnold H. Glasgow

"Strength does not come from physical capacity.
It comes from an indomitable will."
-Mahatma Ghandi

"You must live in the present. Launch yourself on
every wave. Find your eternity in each moment."
-Henry David Thoreau

"If you don't have dream, how are you going
to make a dream come true?"
-Oscar Hammerstein

"Lost wealth may be replaced by industry, lost
knowledge by study, lost health by temperance
or medicine, but lost time is gone forever."
-Samuel Smiles

"Success is not forever and failure isn't fatal."
-Don Shula

"Thank God for competition. When our competitors upset our plans or outdo our designs, they open infinite possibilities of our own work to us."
-Gil Atkinson

"The only thing that stands between a man and what he wants from life is often merely the will to try it and the faith to believe that it is possible."
-Richard M. DeVos

"When you cannot make up your mind which of two evenly balanced courses of action you should take-choose the bolder."
-William Joseph Slim

"If you focus on results, you will never change. If you focus on change, you will get results."
-Jack Dixon

"In the field of observation, chance favors only the prepared minds."
-Louis Pasteur

"I am not judged by the number of times I fall, but by the number of times I succeed; and the number of times I succeed is in direct proportion to the number of times I can fall and keep on trying."
-Tom Hopkins

"We are continuously faced by great opportunities brilliantly disguised as insoluble problems."
-Lee Iacocca

"Life affords no higher pleasure than that of surmounting difficulties, passing from one step of success to another, forming new wishes, and seeing them gratified."
-Samuel Johnson

"If you want to take your mission in life to the next level, if you're sick and you don't know how to rise, don't look outside yourself. Look inside. Don't let your fears keep you mired in the crowd. Abolish your fears and raise your commitment level to the point of no return, and I guarantee you that the Champion Within you burst forth to propel you toward victory."
-Bruce Jenner

"To accomplish great things, we must not only act, but also dream; not only plan, but also believe."
-Anatole France

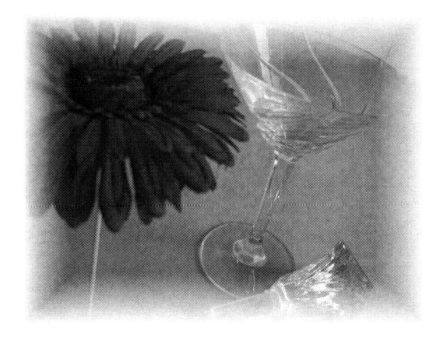

A Feast of Great Thoughts
a.k.a. Smorgasbord

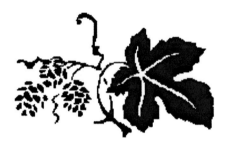

"But we often look so long and so regretfully
upon the closed door that we do not
see the one which has opened for us."
-Helen Keller

"A good plan today is better than
a perfect plan tomorrow."
-General George S. Patton

"The activist is not the man who says the river is dirty.
The activist is the man who cleans up the river."
-Ross Perot

"If you keep thinking about what you want to do
or what you hope will happen, you don't
do it, and it won't happen"
-Joe Dimaggio

"What you get by achieving your goals is not as
important as what you become by achieving your
goals."
-Zig Ziglar

"Circumstances may cause interruptions and delays,
but never lose sight of the goal. Prepare yourself in
every way you can by increasing your knowledge and
adding to your experience, so that you can make the
most of opportunity when it occurs."
-Mario Andretti

"Remember you can't steal second if you
don't take your foot off first."
-Mike Todd

"An adventure is only an inconvenience rightly
considered. An inconvenience is only
adventure wrongly considered."
-G.K. Chesterton

"Nothing is as real as a dream. The world can change
around you, but your dream will not. Responsibilities
need not erase it. Duties need not obscure it.
Because the dream is within
you, no one can take it away."
-Tom Clancy

"You will become as small as your controlling desire,
as great as your dominant aspiration.
-James Allen

"The main dancers in this life are the people who want
to change everything or nothing. "
-Lady Nancy Astor

"You can do anything if your have enthusiasm.
Enthusiasm is the yeast that makes your hopes rise to
the stars. With it, there is accomplishment.
Without it, there are only alibis."
-Henry Ford

"Aim at perfection in everything, though in most things it is unattainable. However, they who aim at it, and persevere, will come much nearer to it than those whose laziness and despondency make them give it up as unattainable."
-Lord Chesterfield

"Always bear in mind that your own resolution to success is more important than any other one thing."
-Abraham Lincoln

"What this power is I cannot say, all I know is that it exists and it becomes available only when a man is in that state of mind in which he knows exactly what he wants and is fully determined not to quit until he finds it."
-Alexander Graham Bell

"My mother said to me, 'If you become a soldier, you'll be a general; if you become a monk, you'll end up as the pope.' Instead, I became a painter and wound up a Pablo Picasso."
-Pablo Picasso

"Success supposes endeavor."
-Jan Austen

"Things may come to those who wait, but only the things left by those who hustle."
-Abraham Lincoln

"The most important single ingredient in the formula of success, is knowing how to get along with people."
-Theodore Roosevelt

"It is only as we develop others that we permanently succeed."
-Harvey S. Firestone

"The world is full of abundance and opportunity, but far too many people come to the fountain of life with a sieve instead of a tank car... a teaspoon instead of a steam shovel. They expect little and as a result they get little."
-Ben Sweetland

"No pessimist ever discovered the secrets of stars, or sailed to an uncharted land, or opened a new heaven to the human spirit."
-Helen Keller

"The expectations of life depend upon diligence; the mechanic that would perfect his work must first sharpen his tools."
-Confucius

"A man who wants to lead the orchestra must turn his back on the crowd."
-Thomas Crook

"As life is action and passion, it is required of a man
that he should share the passion and action of his time,
at peril of being judged not to have lived."
-Oliver Wendell Holmes Jr.

"Entrepreneurs are simply those who understand
that there is little difference between obstacle and
opportunity and are able to turn both to their
advantage."
-Victor Kia

"Confidence doesn't come out of nowhere. It's a result of
something…hours and days and weeks and years
of constant work and dedication."
-Roger Staubach

"Never mistake motion with action."
-Ernest Hemingway

"Have confidence that if you have done a little thing
well, you can do a bigger thing well too."
-David Storey

"To attain happiness in another world, we need only to
believe something; to secure it in this world,
we must do something."
-Charlotte Perkins Gilman

"I place very little value on simplicity that lay on this
side of complicity but a great deal on that
which lay on the other side."
-Olive Wendell Holmes

"Loyalty, friendship, family ties, the duty owed to an ideal – in our time, these obligations seem to have lost their force as motivators and connectors."
-Elizabeth Janeway

"Gratitude makes sense of our past, brings peace for today, and creates a vision for tomorrow."
- Melody Beattie

"What we must decide is perhaps how we are valuable rather than how valuable we are."
- Edgar Z. Friedenberg

"The most luxurious possession, the richest treasure anybody has, is his personal dignity."
-Jackie Robinson

"If you have sincerity, all other things will be added to you."
-A. S. Neill

"Instead of developing your personality, charm, or intellect, try exercising your character today."
- Stephanie Goddard Davidson

"I have to live with myself, and so I want to be fit for myself to know."
-Edgar A. Guest

"You'll never find yourself until you face the truth."
- Pearl Bailey

"Peace is happiness digesting."
- Victor Hugo

"The willingness to accept responsibility for one's own
life is the source from which self-respect springs."
-Joan Didion

"A loving heart is the truest wisdom."
- Charles Dickens

"The wealth of a soul is measured by how much
it can feel, its poverty by how little."
- William R. Alger

"An ambitious man can never know peace."
-J. Krishnamurti

"Character is much easier kept than recovered."
-Thomas Paine

"One's philosophy is not best expressed in words;
it is expressed in the choices one makes."
-Eleanor Roosevelt

"All problems boil down to limited choices,
and the choice we often forget is love."
- Tom Daly

"The truth is, there's no better time to be happy than right
now....Your life will always be filled with challenges."
- Richard Carlson

"If you don't accept failure as a possibility, you don't
set high goals, you don't branch out, you don't try - -
you don't take the risk."
- Rosalynn Carter

"True consistency, that of the prudent and the wise,
is to act in conformity with circumstances."
-John C. Calhoun

"The key to change... is to let go of fear."
- Rosanne Cash

"We'll go dancing, and then we'll do it again."
-Peter Breinholt

"Flops are a part of life's menu and I've never been a
girl to miss out on any of the courses."
- Rosalind Russell

"Opinions are made to be changed –
or how is truth to be got at?"
- Lord Byron

"Life's most persistent and urgent question is:
What are you doing for others?"
- Martin Luther King Jr.

"Every one of us has in himself a continent of
undiscovered character. Happy is he who acts the
Columbus to his own soul."
- Sir J. Stevens

"The only thing that makes one place more attractive to
me than another is the quantity of hearts I find in it."
-Jane Welsh Carlyle

"Habit is overcome by habit."
-Thomas a' Kempis

"Act as if it were impossible to fail."
-Dorothea Brande

"Power is the ability to do good things for others."
- Brooke Astor

"Those who are animated by hope can perform what would seem impossibilities to those who are under the depressing influence of fear."
-Marie Edgeworth

"The best informed man is not always the wisest."
- Dietrich Bonhoeffer

"Chance favors the prepared mind."
- Louis Pasteur

"Ideals are like stars; you will not succeed in touching them with your hands... you choose them as your guides, and following them you will reach your destiny."
- Carl Schultz

"The ideal man bears the accidents of life with dignity and grace, making the best of circumstances."
- Aristotle

"Here's a test to find whether your mission on earth is finished; If you're alive, it isn't..."
- Richard Bach

"An idea in a cage is like a silver dollar buried in the ground. Both are safe, but neither produces anything."
- Dr. Myron S. Allen

"Make it a point to rid your speech and thoughts of all forms of negative self-talk."
- Karl Albrecht

"If a man is often the subject of conversation he soon becomes the subject of criticism."
- Immanuel Kant

"What is really important in education is.. that the mind is matured, that energy is aroused."
- Soren Kierkegaard

"Authority without wisdom is like a heavy axe without an edge, fitter to bruise than polish."
-Anne Bradstreet

"Pursue your passion and live your dream."
- Katherine Logan

"If there is any peace it will come through being, not having."
-Henry Miller

" 'Tis the motive exalts the action;
'Tis the doing, and not the deed."
- Margaret Preston

"I don't want to get to the end of my life and find that I
just lived the length of it. I want to have
lived the width of it as well."
- Diane Ackerman

"The only competition worthy a wise
man is with himself."
-Anna Brownell Jameson

"True friends stab you In the front."
- Oscar Wilde

"To reconstruct is to collaborate with time gone by,
penetrating or modifying its spirit, and
carrying it toward a longer future."
- Marguerite Yourcenar

"Everybody is talented, original and has
something important to say."
- Brenda Ueland

"All I ever wanted....couldn't hold a candle to what I've
been given. I've been given what I need."
- Michael McLean

<u>Afterward</u>

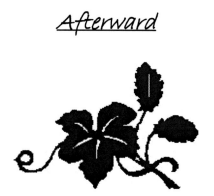

Individuals tend to reach for answers through either their own past experience or through others. Quotes are used on a regular basis in applying experience into modern day challenges and quests. Answers are not found in quotes; quotes simply offer an alternate perspective.

Brain Snacks was created to make the reader think. Every one of us has the opportunity to ponder and consider statements, and apply them to our own personal situations and beliefs. Most of us have a favorite quote or series of quotes. They become part of us without our even realizing it. The way that we use and reference quotes, is a fingerprint of our expression and mindset.

There is not one perfect quote, as that is simply based on opinion. What is unique about using quotes is that they can have numerous meanings. The way an individual uses voice and inflection, can dramatically alter a quote. One quote can have thousands of implications. Quotes can profoundly impact an individual statement, which is why they are commonly used by politicians, mentors, and speakers throughout the world.

Expand your appetite for thought-provoking knowledge!
Enjoy some Brain Snacks!

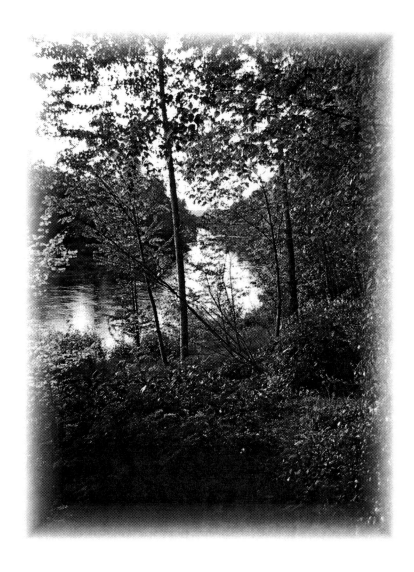

Acknowledgements

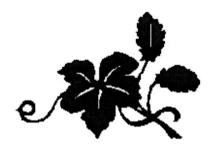

Most goals that individuals aspire to and dream about accomplishing require inspiration, determination, and courage. Believing in oneself is what it takes. However, sometimes that is not enough, and it also takes the encouragement of respected and loved ones in your life to push you to the next level.

For that, I acknowledge all those in my life who push me to be the best I can be; to accomplish goals I never realized I would be setting forth to do; to believe that everything happens for a reason and that there is a time and place for situations to occur.

My gracious thanks extend to those who share my day to day life experiences. You walk with me everywhere I go. I truly believe these individuals, who know whom they are, are the champagne in my life. You bring me joy, show me how effervescent life can be, and allow me to celebrate how lucky I am to have you in my life.

About the Author

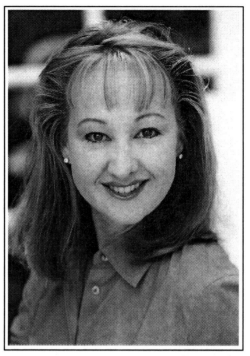

Photo by Paul DaSilva

Shelli Margheritis is the author of "Making The Move;" an IPPY Award nominee. She has worked extensively within the dance and entertainment industry for numerous years, and continues to influence these arenas through her company Solutions, Inc.
Shelli and her husband reside in Southern California.

For additional information check out www.skmsolutions.com.

CPSIA information can be obtained at www.ICGtesting.com
Printed in the USA
LVOW110105281011

252346LV00002B/170/A